The Broken
OPEN Road
To Mental Health

It IS My Business

SHARON FEKETE

Copyright © 2024 Sharon Fekete

No part of this book may be reproduced or transmitted in any form or by any means, electronic or mechanical, including photocopying, recording or by any information storage or retrieval system, without written permission from the author and the publisher, except for the inclusion of a brief quotation in a review.

ISBN: 9798218486518

Rob and Cooper, this one's for you.

I love you.

iv

Contents

Chapter One: The Road Behind; Reflections From Writing My Memoir 1

Chapter Two: Broken Open 9

Chapter Three: St. Bernadette & The Whispers 15

Chapter Four: The Pandemic Pause 23

Chapter Five: Let the Trauma Healing Begin 29

Chapter Six: Whispers through Meditation 35

Chapter Seven: Mental Health in the Workplace 43

Chapter Eight: Where I'm From 51

Chapter Nine: An EAP Saved My Life 59

Chapter Ten: The Deafening Silence 67

Chapter Eleven: Isolation to Community; Reflections on AA 75

Chapter Twelve: HEALERS 83

Chapter Thirteen: Dad, what is this here to teach me? ..91

CHAPTER ONE
The Road Behind; Reflections From Writing My Memoir

'M BACK WHERE it all started five years ago. I chose the exact same day, April 8th, to begin the process and follow the same five-day schedule. Yes, I wrote the last book in five days and my intention is to do the same with this one except *today* there is a solar eclipse scheduled and the moon is in retrograde. What that means exactly as it pertains to this book I have yet to find out. I didn't even know there was a solar eclipse happening today. I only knew this date has been on the calendar since the beginning of 2024. I hadn't even told my husband or anyone really close to me about writing this second book until last night after I visited an intuitive consultant on a whim. It was pretty random for me to get in the car and hope an intuitive consultant was available on a Sunday afternoon for 15 minutes, but she was and here we are, waiting for a solar eclipse and writing my second book documentary style.

I feel most comfortable reporting to you exactly how life is happening at this moment and then I will shift into what has transpired over the last five years. It is pretty outrageous that everyone reading this book across the globe will know exactly what the world has been like since 2020. The year we were all excited about the opportunities of a new decade. I was so pumped that I even booked tickets for the first weekend of January with a girlfriend to see Oprah's 2020 Vision tour: Your Life In Focus. My friend surprised me with an upgrade and we sat (6) rows back from Oprah Winfrey, my idol, and then learned the surprise guest was Lady Gaga! HELLO!! Oprah AND Lady Gaga? I was pumped about 2020 and well, we all know what happened next.

If I'm being completely honest, I'm not as excited to write this book as I was with my memoir. It seems as though it can be a lot easier to write about your previous life than it is to share how much I've changed since putting pen to paper (or actually, fingers to the keyboard). I did not foresee how much work I still had to do on myself until I released book number one, The Broken Road to Mental Health in Life and In Business. Prior to releasing that book in 2019, I thought I was pretty healthy but there was so much work left to be done.

So here I am now, sitting in the exact same room I fondly refer to as "The Tree Room" at my workspace, The Ring, in Clearwater, Florida. When I made the decision to write my memoir in 2019 to commemorate my 25th year of sobriety, I didn't know everything (including the world as we knew it) would change. The only desire I had when writing that book was to help the one person who might be reading it to feel less alone. I didn't have any inkling that one of the people who really needed help was me. I truly didn't know that the book I wrote would in fact save me. The work had only begun and I will do my best to walk you through that unraveling process in this book.

Let's talk about a few key things first that were so incredibly enjoyable when I released The Broken

Road to Mental Health, which going forward will be referred to as TBR2MH. I can only describe it as life changing in every way possible. It brought on some of the most incredible conversations that I would ever have in my life, and it opened me up to a healing I didn't know I needed. It ultimately led others to feeling safe in sharing their most intimate pain with me, a gift I will never take for granted. I received countless letters and private messages from family, friends, and people I have never met to say how my story impacted their lives. There were many that had lost a loved one to suicide or overdose and were brave enough to share their sacred stories with me and ask questions. I saved every message and honor those precious memories that are now deeply locked away in my heart.

I was able to make closer connections within my family that never knew some of the struggles I experienced in my younger years. One in particular that stands out is with my younger brother Sean. To this day, it is one of my most precious memories. After reading the book we had a long conversation about the pain it caused within our family. Even though it hurt to hear of all the pain I inflicted on his young life, we were able to become even closer as a brother and sister. Of course, we shared some great laughter as he informed me that our parents told him I was away in computer school when I was actually in a rehab! It still baffles my mind the amount of pain the entire family endures when living with a loved one that suffers from addiction and depression. I will elaborate more about this matter in later chapters. I also received the most touching phone call from my Godfather, Uncle Martin. He told me how proud he was of me that I put this all down on paper for others to benefit from and that memory will live inside of me for years to come.

Of course there are bittersweet moments with my parents, husband, and stepson that mean more to me than words could ever express. Especially now that my Father was diagnosed with Alzheimer's in 2021 and my Mother-In-Law entered into memory care in 2022. I am grateful that I have documented my Father opening my book and sharing his undying love and pride for the work I've done. I have since recorded my parents openly discussing their reactions and they have provided comfort and solace to those that are entangled in the mess of this family disease. To this day, 30 years later, with significant memory loss, Dad remembers the pain inflicted from my addiction and depression. I will elaborate more in later chapters as we have most recently shared some beautiful moments.

I have learned impactful lessons about the language we use when having conversations surrounding suicide. I didn't know before 2019 that it is best to say "died by suicide" versus "committed suicide." Now I know that the word commit brings us back to a time when suicide was considered a sin or a crime. It took many conversations with educated people in the professional field of mental health to understand why this matters; I recommend you do the same.

After I released my book, I didn't know how to continue the conversation but I knew it needed to happen. I was getting so much feedback about the loneliness and shame surrounding these conversations so I would host small local events for people that read my book. They would come and simply connect with others in a courageous space, and that grew into hosting a podcast. I will take you with me on this documented broken road to mental health and hopefully we will continue to heal together.

8

CHAPTER TWO
Broken Open

LOVE DOCUMENTING LIFE and I'm certain today I got that from my Father. He used to carry around a camera wherever we went and then moved up to one of those gigantic home video cameras. When I walked out of the elevator in my wedding dress Dad had the camera in one hand and he was talking on the phone in the other. It never changed, his love for pictures runs deep in our home and there's a photo gallery of memories thanks to my parents. We have hundreds of unwatched VHS tapes documenting our life and family thanks to Dad.

I have since taken over the reigns and thankfully this documentation process has gotten a lot easier over the years. I have thousands of pictures stored in my phone & there was a time I did a daily vlog on YouTube, I stopped when I hit 300 videos. I actually just watched the daily vlog I did after writing my last book & happy to report so far, this one isn't as traumatizing. Which leads to the actual name of this book, The Broken OPEN Road to Mental Health. These last 5 years have in fact broken me right open and it all started by writing my memoir.

There was an enormous amount of time spent at the Hilton on Clearwater Beach before and after I wrote my book. I have so many pictures and videos documenting the experience. As mentioned, the only goal was to help one person so I also recorded the entire book on my podcast at the Hilton before professionally recording it on Audible. It's still there for free on The Doctor Whisperer podcast if you want to hear the AC unit in the room and pigeons in the background. It was VERY raw but I'm grateful I have that so I never forget how life changing this moment in time was for me. I listened to Lauren Daigle to help me heal and cried for hours alone while the trauma I endured slowly began to leave my body.

The first physical reaction I had to witnessing the trauma leaving my body was present during a massage at the Hibiscus Spa. I had booked my parents into the same hotel to celebrate the upcoming release of my book and Mom was enjoying a spa day with me. I had been crying uncontrollably as the beautiful therapist held space for me through my tears. When I got back to meet Mom in the relaxation room she was consoling me and I vividly remember telling her I would never be the same again. I don't know if Mom could grasp at that moment what I meant, but I knew in my soul, life was about to take a big turn.

Writing my book was like an out of body experience while remaining IN my body! I never took into account how painful it could be to relive those terrifying events I had endured as an active alcoholic/addict. I took it for granted that I had been sober for all those years and I was "good" now. Writing that book forced me to face those traumatic moments that I had suppressed for so long. I spent 25 years of my life in 12-step recovery focusing on the solution and pushing down the trauma I survived. Writing the book offered many sleepless nights and the quiet meditation was replaced with guided meditation, as my thoughts were so intrusive. I was faced with memories coming back to life that I had pushed down for decades.

There was no way of knowing that a true healing was about to walk into my life and it started with my book and that massage at the Hilton. I was about to uncover how much work I still had to do and will remain doing for the rest of my life. I will get to that trauma healing later but for now, I want to shed some more light on this experience. I was sober 25 years and had never faced the horrific events that happened to me as a 19 year old that blacked out and moved to Detroit from NY. Please take a moment to consider what can happen to a young blackout drinker that was high daily until she turned 21 years old and moved back home. I joked for 25 years as I told my story in AA that I blacked out and woke up in Detroit, but it's actually not funny. It's a miracle I'm alive and have lived to tell my story, so now I would like share some serious awakenings with you.

Let's start with what the physician told me after I got sober and learned I was suicidal. This Psychiatrist told me that I had a chemical imbalance and I needed to start taking Prozac. In my book, I almost gleefully reported this information to you because after 25 years of sobriety and freedom from depression with NO medication, I still believed I had a chemical imbalance. Can you see the insanity in all of this? If it wasn't for my EAP (Employee Assistance Program) counselor, Ben, I might still be medicated today. (see first book for more about my journey with Ben) DISCLAIMER: I am 100% **not** opposed to medication; I am opposed to bullshit though. Believe me, I am still grateful I was offered 20mg of Prozac because I believe it was absolutely necessary to get me back on track but a **chemical imbalance**? Forget about the doctor, how come I never questioned this statement? The logic of it all today makes me so irritated. I had not taken medication in all these years yet I believed the story a doctor told me. AARGH! I said it to rooms of people for 25 years and actually believed it to be true.

I can honestly say if I didn't read the book Lost Connections by Johann Hari after releasing my book I might never have learned about the bullshit that is out there in the world of medical marketing. I am also eternally grateful for the work and writings of Dr. Gabor Mate on trauma, it saved me these last five years. Knowing that trauma is not what happened TO me, it's what happened inside of me brings me to tears even writing this now. I will elaborate more on my healing journey in chapter 5 but for now I wanted you to know why I **had** to write a follow-up book. Yes, a sober woman of many years can live in the dark and trauma can seep out in other ways. I know, it has happened to me and I can clearly see all the patterns today.

Now that we've gotten the deeper meaning behind the title of the book, let me tell you how it actually came to be. I've discussed the whispers before and this one was loud and clear while running up the Belleair Causeway a few months ago. I was getting my morning inspiration listening to Oprah's Super Soul podcast and my sports bra popped wide open! Yes, I had a shirt on too but was flappin' around in the wind and just burst out laughing at myself. I was at the top of the bridge knowing I had to walk back down and glanced at the name of the episode I was listening to and boom, "Broken Open." You just can't make this shit up, and hence, the title of this book!

CHAPTER THREE

St. Bernadette & The Whispers

WROTE THIS BLOG on the platform Medium on April 17th, 2020 and I thought it was appropriate to include in this book. Please read below and I will follow up with comments as they apply today in 2024. I can't help but say that this chapter title makes me think of a name to a band. Not a band I would see, but just want to keep you as close to the way my mind operates as possible throughout this book.

Let me start by saying... I'm not one to talk about saints and churches. I have been on a spiritual journey for 25 years now and I believe a strong force lives inside all of us. I'm also promising not to think too hard about what I'm about to share because if I do I might not make it through this blog. I'm just going to tell you a story of what happened to me in October of 2019.

I released my first book, The Broken Road to Mental Health, in Life and in Business on August 11th, 2019. That was the day of my 25th sober anniversary, also known as my Mom's birthday. On October 10th, 2019, I celebrated my 10 year wedding anniversary & then my 47th birthday on October 13th. So, just to frame it up....there was a lot going on. (I'm also a stepmom, have 2 fur-babies and own 2 businesses, just sayin...for context).

Some friends of Bill W. (look up reference if you want) invited me to join them on a spiritual retreat, the weekend of October 18th. My first reaction was HELL TO THE NO but that is my natural rebellious reaction internally most days. I was tired, busy, and not in the mood to be around a bunch of people quite honestly at a place run by monks to meditate. I went to a Catholic school and the whole retreat thing at a place called St. Leo's seemed a little much for me at the time. Let me be clear, I love all things spiritual but my plate was full and the last thing I needed was rest. (insert a peak into the brain of an entrepreneur) I was gifted an energy clearing session already & stayed at my "retreat" spot at the Hilton on Clearwater Beach for 3 days so I was 'good.'

Yes, I ended up going. I have been practicing 'opposite action' for about 25 years now. I do the opposite of what my mind initially tells me because I believe the universe has something bigger in store for me. Considering I escaped death a few times I realize my initial decisions might not actually be the best ones.

So…. the wonderful group of people attending this retreat encouraged me to visit 'the grotto' on Saturday night. Initial thought, NO. So I go and everyone is so excited to share in this sacred place & pointing out all of the beautiful statues of Mary, Joseph and other peeps but THIS one featured at the top immediately grabs my attention. I am going to report exactly what happened…now…

I turned to this statue behind me and immediately thought, "what the hell happened to you?" She looked so sad…desperate….in pain. I asked her what happened and then I took her picture. I leaned back a SKOSH and took another picture.

(notice, she's looking right at me with a different 'look'…keep going back and forth between the pictures and TELL ME how her neck turned and looked at me like that!!) She told me she needed my help. That's what she said. She needed my help…I'm crying as I write this now because it was so powerful and so abundantly clear. I never shared what she said with anyone but THAT is what she SAID!! I understood what she meant then and I understand it today even more on a very deep level.

I asked the monks at breakfast the next morning who she was and I was told it was St. Bernadette. I was kind of bummed that it wasn't St. Theresa…it would have made more sense. Or so I thought… she needed my help and wanted me to keep speaking up about mental health, depression, addiction, alcoholism, and offer HOPE to others. That's what she wanted. She knew of the break in tradition I believed I was making within my 12 step community but she set me free that day. Too many people need help right now and I need to be ok with offending people. It has been an internal struggle to a degree that I could never actually put into words. A decision to stay radically vulnerable outside of my recovery rooms.

I had no plan. I didn't intend on writing that book in 2019, it wasn't on my 2019 goals list (I write business goals at the end of every year). That book came through me, not out of me. I wanted to offer hope to all of those that may think they are alone. I wanted to encourage others in the business community to come apart and still be strong. To extend an offering that might not be 'the popular' thing to do...but the right thing. I was set free the moment I made the decision to live a life that was saved so many times before.

It turns out St. Bernadette was pretty badass! She had many believers and a ton of skeptics. Her life was pretty miserable until Mary spoke to her in Lourdes, France at the grotto. Ironically, considering today's temporary new normal, she died from complications of pulmonary issues. Maybe irony isn't the right sentiment so let's just call it grace.

Mary spoke to Bernadette and then she spoke to me. I called Mom before I wrote this blog to see if she still had a picture of me crowning the Virgin Mary after my 1st Communion. Mom wanted to carry out an Irish tradition in East Rockaway, NY and I was to crown the Virgin Mary (can you see the image of an innocent 2nd grader in her communion dress crowning the Virgin Mary and then a few years later moving to Detroit in a blackout?!). Not sure if I was too thrilled about the "May Procession to Church" then but I am certainly connecting some spiritual dots here now! I remember holding that rosary tight and crowning Mary on that windy day in Long Island like it was yesterday.

Today is the Feast of St. Bernadette. I believe in my heart she is watching over all of us now. I also believe when she was taken to that mental asylum because of her convictions that she was yet another mental health warrior. It's yet another whisper to keep on going…to never give up…to keep sharing hope with others…to live a life of service….this too shall pass.

So, just one week ago from writing this book, Mom was showing me old photos of my communion again. The dress meant something very deep to my Mom. She has showed me this picture a few times in my life and is sure to point out the details of the dress each time. Feels like a whisper. (if you know you know)

I have recently stumbled upon the teachings of Dr. Peter Levine, developer of the Somatic Experiencing approach. Trauma studies reveal that suffering and unhappiness are often passed on to future generations and can hold a powerful influence over our emotions and behaviors today, usually without us ever knowing why. Dr. Levine has uncovered methods to help separate us from the transgenerational pain that stunts our future growth. I am currently captivated by my ancestors' suffering and how that transcends through generations. Not in a morbid way but more out of a curiosity that will continue to help us stop passing on generational trauma. Maybe by the next book, I will have discovered even more about this 'whisper' I received in the grotto that day. For now, I think it is worth your time to look up Dr. Levine's work if you want to learn more.

Since we have yet to uncover my pandemic pause, I will briefly mention that I had an opportunity to interview best selling Author, Lorna Byrne. She's an Irish author who's been seeing angels since she was a child. I highly doubt there is any coincidence that I was to interview her on The Broken Road to Mental Health podcast. Serendipity brought me to her NYC publicist and connected us for this divine engagement. Lorna told me that St. Bernadette had been many whispers all through my life & that I resembled her. She said, "It's almost like you're connected to her family, her sister in a way." She told me that the communion crowning was all part of the journey.

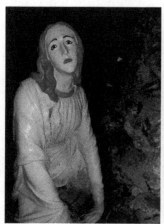
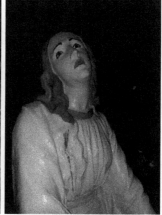

CHAPTER FOUR
The Pandemic Pause

WE CERTAINLY DIDN'T see a pandemic coming in our 2019 countdown to 2020! It's hard to believe four years have gone by since we were all sequestered to our homes and an entire new language and new world started to take shape. Isolation, the new normal, transmission, quar antine, social distancing, fatality rate, collective grief, ventilator, rising death tolls, racial reckoning, burnout, collective trauma, zoom, work from home, hybrid model, pivot, Instacart, curbside, TikTok, remote work, in-person, virtual conference, banning books, Roe V Wade overturned, insurrection…I now simply refer to it as global trauma.

This previous paragraph was tough to type & even harder to live through so let's please take a breath before we continue…

How did we get through all of this? How did YOU get through all of this? Are you OK? Did you lose someone to COVID? Did you lose a loved one to overdose? Did you lose someone to suicide? Was your loved one in an ALF and were you waving to them from outside? Those images will never leave my mind.

Well, so far this chapter sucks. I went back to my documentation of March 2020, before we were told to stay home to see what was happening in my world. Ironically, I went back to therapy via Teledoc for the first time on March 6th of 2020, days prior to the shutdown. As I previously mentioned, I love documenting the journey so of course I recorded that session and yes, I told the therapist. I only stayed w/ him for a few weeks, we weren't a fit but I am more fascinated with the fact I insinuated that I didn't really need therapy because I was sober 25 years. HOLY SHIT, WTF!

Yes, even after writing my book, The Broken Road to Mental Health in Life and in Business, I thought the answers to my mental health journey solely lived in the solution provided in the rooms of Alcoholics Anonymous. Of course daily exercise, meditation, community, and a solid nutrition plan certainly helped but I implied "I was good." I will elaborate more on how this has since all changed for me in Chapter 13 but for now, I'm taking a moment to honor the pandemic pause. As horrific and traumatizing as many of those days hearing of all the death and destruction while delivering food to my parents house so they didn't get sick, I'm grateful for the pause.

This pause changed everything for me and I hope it did for you too. The change was slow but has continued to evolve as the years tick off the clock. I want to first share what I now realize, I was the young girl not yet healed from her trauma doing everything she could to help everyone else but herself. First, I made a decision to do a daily podcast show on The Doctor Whisperer platform. I have so many healers in my life and I felt so paralyzed by the helplessness that I did what I could offer at that moment. Then in 2021, I started a weekly podcast show on The Broken Road to Mental Health platform. I couldn't bare to think about the newcomers trying to get sober and having no in-person meetings so I started a

Saturday Zoom meeting. I was suicidal when I stopped drinking and drugging and "isolation" was the thing I needed to avoid most so I felt called to take action. Since I was now being more open about discussing mental health, I called it 'Recovery Journey to Mental Wellness' and it is in fact an AA meeting that still runs on Saturday's. I have since passed the baton after 4 years and will forever believe in the spirit of rotation. My dear friend Nancy brought a pamphlet to my attention that was printed in 2018 called AA for Alcoholics with Mental Health Issues and we read it together every Saturday morning at 8am.

Believe me, I almost wish I was bragging about all the things I did to offer service, but it simply exposes a woman who has yet to resolve her traumatic past.

Just to stay on brand for another minute, I also started a completely different 2nd book in April of 2020 while running 2 businesses in a pandemic. It was more of a companion book to the first one with daily quotes, thoughts reflecting the quote, and of course a business tip at the end. I made it through April 30th and then my therapist Sam suggested I take a break. WHY? Well, because I was taking quotes from people that had died by suicide and/or overdose. Then I would go down massive rabbit holes to try and understand what happened to them. Imagine if you will, the state of the world in April of 2020 and my decision to write that book. WHAT was going on?

I mentioned a therapist, well, that's what saved the day and stopped me from this vicious cycle. Thankfully I didn't give up on my hunt for a great therapist after the first one in March of 2020 and Sam and I have since done a lot of work together these last few years. I will elaborate on more of the healing later but I am forever grateful for the incredible work of therapists today. In certain circles now they even refer to me as the therapy pusher, a title that brings much pride.

Sam and I realized together there was much work to be done and a lot of it revolved around avoiding conflict to maintain harmony. I had so much unresolved trauma that needed to be addressed and healed. Although I am forever humbled so many people shared how my memoir helped them, it ultimately saved me.

I would like to add that I'm thrilled to share this news with you today. Even though I was sober 25 years when I published my book, I thought I was a pretty healthy gal. I am not bitter at all about the time it has taken to gain this sense of knowing and clarity. In fact, I believe it is all in divine order. I do not think I would have been as receptive as I am to it now. Dare I say, I don't believe my fragile brain and heart would have been strong enough to endure opening up this part of my life at 21 years old. At 51 and (3) decades away from the life I survived, I also believe I am nowhere near done healing. I am certainly healthier than I've ever been in my mind and my body today but there is more work to be done. I have learned so much about myself and that little girl I never wanted to revisit. The one who endured so much pain and trauma yet some higher source saw fit to send a few cranes along the way to lift me out of the rubble.

CHAPTER FIVE
Let the Trauma Healing Begin

*"Trauma is not what happens to you,
trauma is what happens inside you."*
-Dr. Gabor Mate

LOVE LISTENING TO Audible books. I'm also a big fan that the algorithm understands exactly what book to recommend next. It's almost like Audible really wants me to get healthier, shout out to you Bezos! The first book I listened to after I released my memoir was The Awakened Woman by Dr. Tererai Trent. She told me to bury my sacred dreams in the dirt and to be courageous, not silent. I needed to hear that message because there was an inner critic telling me not to continue down this path. Today my sacred dreams are buried in my backyard thanks to the help of Rob and Cooper, as they helped & were witness to the burial. I will be sure to share these sacred dreams with you soon as they have already started to come true.

The next book that popped up was the one previously mentioned in Chapter 2, Lost Connections, by Johann Hari. I can honestly tell you that this one made me rethink my entire life and helped unravel the story I was telling myself for 25 years. The line under the title grabbed me, 'uncovering the real causes of depression and the unexpected solutions.' I have listened to this book at least 5 times and I refer back to it often when speaking about mental health in the workplace. I was about to learn why I suffered from depression, 25 years later.

I could not recommend this book more to anyone who wants to understand why they're depressed or why their loved one is struggling. Johann has done extensive research with some of the most acclaimed physicians across the globe. His work has an enormous amount of data to support the information in the book and considering I've worked with doctors for over 20 years now, I really understand the broken 'system.' There certainly is a crack in the old story and I'm so grateful I was able to read this and change mine.

I have written extensively about my Dad's EAP (employee assistance program) counselor that saved my life by asking "are you having suicidal thoughts?" I was then brought to said Psychiatrist that told me I had a chemical imbalance and this Prozac would help. It did, but today I believe it was mostly placebo because if you give a drug to a drug addict, it will help. It absolutely gave me courage in a pill form that I needed to keep showing up to therapy and attending my AA meetings. There were probably even more benefits that I'm unaware of today but if it wasn't for my therapist guiding me along the weaning process, I could still be medicated today. I got lucky. I had someone who knew it was going to take more than a pill to pull me out of my suicidal thoughts. He insisted I regularly attend 12 step meetings and get involved in the community. Ben knew I needed the support of people who could identify with the pain of addiction and my group of friends certainly saved my life. I received what a lot of people do not when alcoholism and addiction cross their path, the RIGHT guidance.

All that aside, the doctor told me I had a chemical imbalance in my brain and I told that story to everyone that would listen for 25 years. It's even in my book! I learned reading (listening) to Johann's book that this mantra of "chemical imbalance" is repeated in doctor's offices, medical textbooks and obviously in pharmaceutical advertisements. The only problem, and it's a DOOZIE, is that this explanation isn't true. Without having any clinical experience myself I can easily see how stupid it was that I believed this and I haven't had a chemical in my body for almost 30 years now. How on EARTH could I have a chemical imbalance if I only took 20mg's of Prozac for six months? It is infuriating to type these words today, especially knowing what I know now.

Before I go any further I feel like I'm an actual walking disclaimer at all times. By no uncertain terms does this mean I am against medication; it just means **I** was fed a line of bullshit. As a matter of fact, if YOU told me Prozac didn't save my life before writing my first book, I might have been obliged to punch you dead in your neck. So there's that. I believed the story I was told and now I don't.

Then in walks Dr. Gabor Mate to my AirPods. I was listening to a podcast I love called "Last Day" in January of 2020 and lost my shit. I heard him say "Trauma is not what happens to you, trauma is what happens inside you." W H A T?????? You mean to tell me that the trauma I endured as a young adult has been living inside of me for 25 years and led me to that depression when I was 21? NOW I'm finding out the reason I spent so many years of my life in dysfunctional relationship dynamics, assuming the role of the giver and sacrificing my own needs and well-being for the sake of the takers in my life?!

W H A T???? I was getting an education of a lifetime by listening to books and podcasts and then back to therapy I went.

I started talking about the trauma I endured as a young addicted girl lost in Detroit, Michigan. My therapist was kind enough to read my book before we started so I could catch him up to date on who I was before these revelations. We met frequently in the beginning and now I go in for a tune-up every other month. I needed those sessions and we were able to isolate a lot of the patterns I needed to break. Especially when it comes to sacrificing my own needs for others and I had decades of unconscious behaviors to unpack. My nervous system became accustomed to not only tolerating chaos, but feeling a sense of control within it. Hence why I found myself in so many dysfunctional relationships over the years and remained in toxic workplaces while seeking out friends who were takers versus givers.

This continued to unravel until about 2021. I started really working on practicing boundaries and shifting away from relationships in life and in business that were no longer serving me. I have moonwalked out of most relationships that no longer serve me. It has taken a long time to believe I deserve true happiness and that comes with a lot of accountability and practice. I look forward to sharing with you in the next chapter about what has helped me the most these last few years. An unexpected free release of so much internal struggle was just around the corner.

CHAPTER SIX
Whispers through Meditation

THIS NEW YORKER has traveled a lengthy path to finally be broken open by the power of meditation. I am realizing now how much resistance was placed on modalities introduced to my life over thirty years ago. There is a sense of grace flowing through me as I understand there was a divine order placed for this journey. As a sober woman in 12-step recovery, I was introduced to prayer and meditation in the 11th step of AA in my 1st rehab when I was 18 years old. "Sought through prayer and meditation to improve our conscious contact with God as we understand Him, praying only for the knowledge of His will for us and the power to carry that out." Born and raised Catholic, prayer was nothing new to me and I have never resisted a higher source in my life. Today, like many of us, I seek spirituality over religion but have no opinions on what brings someone closer to their source.

I can honestly say I did not practice any kind of meditation until I was 43 years old and working with a client in South Tampa. Ironically, I was introduced to this woman via Valley Bank who was married to a physician. I say "ironically" because Valley Bank to this day has been my biggest corporate supporter of my work surrounding mental health in the workplace. Back then, I was deeply engaged as a consultant for physicians through my business, The Doctor Whisperer. They were about to embark on a space called Evolve Personal Health, combining Eastern and Western modalities, my favorite! Chitra called me and I distinctly remember thinking WHO IS THIS WOMAN? We had an instant connection and I'm proud to tell you that I am still banking with Valley and remain friends with this incredible couple today. Chitra and Vim were creating a space called Evolve Personal Health and I was delighted every day to work with these wonderful people. Chitra was always so grounded and I am definitely attracted to this kind of energy. She is sophisticated, intelligent, but most of all calm. Nothing ever seemed to rock her and I needed to know more. Vim was always smiling and loved to share his healing gifts with practical resources. The whole family, including their daughter Uma, radiated a vibe that's beyond description. I wanted to embody their principles; they truly left a mark on my life forever.

They were destined to broaden the scope of their business and settle in Chicago, but not without profoundly influencing me by the way they conducted their lives. I should also mention they developed a close bond with my parents and ultimately ended up including them in their research and development. We've all enjoyed meals, karaoke, and have reached the heartfelt milestone where my parents have met theirs.

Basically, they ruined me. I began to find it difficult to work with people who didn't share the same vision and convey the type of goodness that lived inside of them. I have since gone on to dissolve The Doctor Whisperer and have also limited the work I offer through my media company to consulting. Today, I have redesigned my business model to attract only those that live in a state of flow. In other words, I learned a lot from them and also continue to evolve.

I first began to incorporate active meditation into my cycling routine, pausing during rides to sit in stillness with a timer set for roughly three minutes. At the time, it was really the longest I could sit in silence. I would eventually discover that it was in fact possible to let thoughts enter my mind and then gently release them. I would gradually practice 5 minutes, and then 10, and 20 became my daily sweet spot. The active meditation moved to incorporating after my exercise routine at home. I would lay on my yoga mat and enjoy the silence before starting my day. This would eventually come to a screeching hault during the pandemic. The noise of the world removed my ability to sit in comfortable silence so I began following guided meditations. It was a wonderful solution and I cried many tears from the pain of the world and then cried tears of joy again for the lessons learned through the pause.

I convinced myself for so many years that my

brain was too busy to slow down and I've also enjoyed throwing in the NYer excuse. If anyone dared ask me about meditation I would quickly say, "I can't sit in silence." Writing that now makes me feel sad because I was telling myself a story that simply wasn't true. The underlying truth was I couldn't stand my own thoughts. Subconsciously I knew how loud it was up in my brain and I simply wasn't ready to get still. I do believe that the limited amount of time I was able to commit in the beginning was linked to the trauma I had yet to heal. There have been many negative conversations with myself through the years and it's only in this last few that I've been able to quiet the noise. Hence why it's called a practice. It certainly didn't happen overnight and I'm still learning more every day.

Today I look forward to meditating as opposed to the torture I once thought it would inflict on my brain. I realize how powerful it is to control our thoughts and now I strive for the ultimate goal, the ability not to react. HOW does Deepak Chopra do it? I was listening to Oprah's podcast interview with him in 2022 when I learned the powerful acronym

STOP. Stop, take a breath, observe my thoughts, and proceed with kindness. This achievement at one time felt so out of reach but today I know it's attainable if I keep working at it. I can already see a difference but I'm definitely a work in progress.

I am lucky enough to work with an incredible client today that listened to the whispers and opened OM Meditation and Wellness right here in Tampa Bay Florida. As I remain in a state of flow, these clients are brought to me and we ultimately develop a relationship that far exceeds these business endeavors. I have thoroughly enjoyed the benefits of group meditation in these silk aerial hammocks and many whispers come to life while floating in the sacred space. Today, I attribute all of my creative ideas to the practice of meditation, walks in nature, good nutrition and cycling. This lifestyle medicine has brought incredible clarity to my world and continues to be vital for my entrepreneurial journey. Meditation helps manage my stress, sharpens my focus, and improves my decision-making. Additionally, it contributes to improving leadership, interpersonal relationships, and helps me navigate the ups and downs of my always-evolving business ventures.

I know today the crane picked me up again and slowly dropped me into meditation. It waited patiently while I prepared myself to sit in silence without replaying the trauma I endured as a young adult. I was ready and the teachers appeared.

> *If you want to change the world, start with yourself.*
>
> *—Mahatma Gandhi*

CHAPTER SEVEN
Mental Health in the Workplace

IF YOU READ my first book you know I added a business parallel and business tip at the end of every chapter. At first I didn't know how I was going to associate my journey through addiction and depression with the world of business but it turns out there were an unfortunate amount of parallels. I was meeting leaders in businesses that were less than honest and riddled with personal drama. I've sadly encountered many affairs, dishonesty, ego, dysfunction, poor leadership, deception, lack of communication and too many traumatized employees. Hosting a reality show based on what I've witnessed would 100% get incredible ratings. The amount of unprofessional professionals out there lurking in the businesses you frequent would shock you.

One of the numerous factors that led me to cease reconstructing medical practices was the overwhelming sadness I felt for the employees. If I were to isolate it to one thing, it was mostly the shock I felt surrounding the lack of communication from leadership. I could walk in and meet with 30 employees and have a full understanding why the business wasn't thriving. It all seemed so simple yet there was a tremendous amount of blame, victimhood, and lack of leadership living in the walls of these businesses. In full transparency, I was disgusted by the end of my days. Especially because I knew the person who was going to pay the ultimate price of these toxic behaviors were the patients.

Opening a media company while consulting for doctors was more of the same. It wasn't as dramatic since there wasn't as much face-to-face time but there was still an incredible amount of inappropriate behavior. To paint a small picture I once had a client that required this exact email response: "My Father doesn't speak to me like this, nor does my husband so I am absolutely NOT going to allow this from you. I will be in my office waiting for your apology." I have had client's wives reach out to my staff and degrade their work that sadly resulted in terminating long-term relationships, and so much more. The most disappointing was a married political figure who stood as a beacon of hope for others in our mental health community hitting on me. I was beginning to understand that I could only make a dent in the work I was doing locally, and I ultimately wanted to make a larger impact.

This was going to take yet another shift in my business life. I dissolved The Doctor Whisperer and decided to primarily focus my business on mental health in the workplace. I've always had a passion to help the masses so I threw my hat in the ring to become a keynote speaker. Serendipitously (it's a thing) I met my speaker coach on one of the podcasts I was hosting at the time. He's known as The Mental Health Comedian, which was perfect since my style has always been laced with humor. I had already delivered many speaking events at medical conferences about hospitality in healthcare and talks surrounding social media, but I wanted to specifically discuss mental health in the workplace.

Hiring an expert that was already actively doing this seemed to make good business sense, and I worked with Frank for an entire year.

How could I have predicted the level of difficulty it would be to pitch a keynote named; "Does Mental Health Live in Your Workplace?" I'm not asking "Does Mental ILLNESS Live in Your Workplace" I'm asking if mental HEALTH lives in your workplace. After I secured my first keynote, I got an email from the organization to see if we could change the title of my talk. This was after signing a contract, developing the speech, and creating the slideshow. **One week** before the conference, this arrived in my inbox; Is there any chance you could revise your title so it doesn't focus so heavily on mental health?

Too bad we can't include a representation of dead silence in a book, please refer to the Audible version for the dramatics. Anyway, I took a deep breath, put my laptop down, and cried. I knew if I said yes to this request, I would be denying a greater purpose. It reminds me of this great quote by one of my faves;

"Daring leaders say the unsaid, unsurface what's been pushed down, and bring to light the stuff that's in the shadows and in the corners."

-Brene Brown

I took some time to breathe and gather my thoughts before sending this response:

Hi,

I attached my signed proposal with the title, "Does Mental Health Live in Your Workplace?". One week before delivering this talk & requesting this change is challenging b/c of my actual work purpose....it is in fact a HIGHER purpose. One of the biggest problems today (and there is a ton of data to support this) is the fear of saying the words mental health...it's the same as physical health and it's a huge problem in the workplace.

I am happy to change it to Mental Health & Wellness in the Workplace with the summary to include Addressing & Overcoming Staff Burnout since my talk will absolutely have a large focus on staff burnout.

I would really like to come to a resolution that works best for all of us but I 100% have your members in mind…. we are ready for a talk with MENTAL HEALTH in the title…and quite honestly, we need it.

Sincerely,

Sharon

PS- I am happy to schedule a conversation or zoom to discuss further. When I flew to Alabama to deliver my last talk for the executive retreat, I got a lot of positive feedback; did you have a different experience?

We ultimately settled on 'Mental Health in the Workplace: Tackling the Tough Conversations.' I delivered my keynote and received an overwhelmingly positive response. My beloved husband sat in the audience and he was able to witness the impact of vulnerable conversations in a business setting. The most satisfying part of delivering my story is the private conversations held when I'm off the stage. I am consistently met with stories of heartache and traumas people have endured. They feel a sense of safety with someone like me who's traveled a broken road. I am able to offer them hope and resources that were readily available to me. It will forever be worth standing in my truth, even if roadblocks continue to present themselves. When it comes to the workplace, we offer a bigger opportunity to help more people. If leaders are trained on how to start these conversations, we will ultimately normalize the words mental health and I won't be asked to change the titles anymore.

CHAPTER EIGHT

Where I'm From

WAS OFFERED AN incredible opportunity from my previous speaker coach to present a talk on a platform called SPEAK. This organization was born from a need to provide a different type of speaking platform for people with ideas and stories. SPEAK talks are 6-10 minutes in length and are delivered in a storytelling format. There are three key moments in a SPEAK talk; the moment of truth, the moment of transformation, and the moment of impact. The theme of the event I was to deliver my talk was HERITAGE, and how it truly shapes who we are and who we have become. The best and scariest part was that it was going to be hosted in my hometown of Long Island, NY. Remember when I mentioned serendipity in business? Well, here we go again. I was introduced to the producer Dana who worked with my sponsor of 28 years, Cynthia, and was cousins with Betsy, who I worked with at NY Medical in my late 20's.

Basically, I was more scared to do this than my first keynote the previous month. I have never been one to memorize anything, I'm more of a 'speak from the heart' kind of girl but this was a challenge I felt compelled to conquer. So after my keynote I went right to work on practicing and memorizing this 8 minute talk. I was excited about the opportunity to share how everyone approaches me after a corporate event and says "Where I'm From, Nobody Talks About Mental Health." The talk was born from every private conversation I've ever had with those beautiful souls who were brave enough to share the mutual silence surrounding shame with me.

Although some very dear friends joined the crowd to witness my talk in my hometown, the only family member in the audience was my brother Sean. I certainly didn't hide the fact that I was speaking in Long Island at this event, I shared it all over social media, but as my Dad always says…."HOWANEVER." Loosely translated from this made up Irish slang, WHATEVS! Probably best since I was incredibly nervous that I was going to forget those (3) key moments of impact. I was also met with some pretty bad news the day before from beloved family matters. How could they have known I was purposely spending the night before in a hotel to meditate, exercise, and deliver my talk with complete clarity the following day? They couldn't attend but I'm positive they would have been there if it wasn't for other obligations.

It just so happens I have the transcript of my talk that I will now leave you with to read. This is also helpful if you didn't read my first book, it's an 8-minute summary of my past life.

Where I'm From, We Don't Talk About Mental Health

"I'm from a residential area".. that's what I told the counselor at the halfway house when I was 19 years old. She told me I would be back if I left Against Medical Advice but I was so depressed and removed from thinking at NINETEEN that I was an alcoholic and knew I would never end up like "these people" b/c I was from a residential area.

"These people" were homeless, heroin addicts, and one woman had AIDS. I grew up in Long Island New York. Born to Irish immigrant parents with 2 brothers…Mom had 12 brothers and Dad had 7 siblings ….yes, we're Irish. I went to private catholic schools, excelled academically and a pretty good athlete until I wasn't. I was very conscious of how I looked and hormones brought body dismorphia and acne to town. Spent most weekends sippin nips in the parking lot of the Commuters Club in East Rockaway…same place my large Irish family were members …the place where many a sing-song took place. Even though we were raised in Long Island, my house was actually IN Ireland. Just because I was mandated to a halfway house after (2) rehabs didn't actually mean I was an alcoholic. I just drank a little too much… WHERE I'M FROM, everyone drinks. I'm Irish.

After a few suicide attempts I went to some of those Alcoholics Anonymous meetings everyone was recommending…then I blacked out and woke up in Detroit, Michigan. To this day I'll never understand why I didn't choose like the Bahamas or somewhere warm … but there I was …Detroit,

Michigan. The only good thing was nobody there knew WHERE I WAS FROM…they didn't know about the rehabs or that sing-song loving Irish family back in the residential area …turns out it doesn't actually matter where you're from when you're homeless and addicted. So I woke up (or 'came to') with a guy named Spokaine…actually it was his alias not a nickname. I eventually left him for Bear, full name Sugar Bear…yes, another alias. He just got out of Jackson State Penitentiary after doing 11 years for kingpen drug dealing. I didn't even know what that was but I was oddly attracted to it.

I was bartending at Brents Place, the sign outside read "where the friendly people meet." Everyone there had a nickname too (wink wink). After that final beating from Bear, I knew it was time to go back to WHERE I'M FROM. Back to the love, safety, innocence and security of my family in Long Island.

When I got back to NY I wanted to die more than I wanted to live …I had no more medicine to take…drugs and alcohol nearly killed me. So I went to the REAL place where the friendly people meet called Alcoholics Anonymous and nobody cared WHERE I CAME FROM … they were just happy I was there and told me to keep coming back. I found my people … my tribe…a group of human beings that discuss the good bad and the ugly while learning how to become better humans on a daily basis. I'm sober 28 years now and hope to never forget where I came from.

I got a REAL toxic job and worked my way up to Director of Operations for a large healthcare practice that eventually went bankrupt. I then decided to move to Florida when I found out my boyfriend had a girlfriend. Yep. Traumatized recovering alcoholic moves to FL and finds a new toxic medical practice to manage. Turns out I was overqualified to manage all this drama but my trauma was really ATTRACTED to the drama. That's the sneaky thing… it will seep out in many ways until you heal from it. Turns out hurt people really DON'T hurt people when they heal.

So…after 8 years managing THIS toxic medical practice filled choc full of affairs and a PIPE BOMB… I opened my own medical consulting company, a small media company and then authored a memoir in 2019. Far beneath that silver lining of the pandemic, I came home to myself. I began another healing from the trauma I endured as a young adult and today I speak about mental health in the workplace. These traumas ooze out when we don't heal...into our relationships, toxic work environments, and family life. What I hear MOST when I leave the stage is "WHERE I'M FROM" nobody talks about mental health, alcoholism, addiction, depression, and suicide. I've heard this from people across the globe, across generations, and across all races and cultures. And yes... WHERE I'M FROM we don't talk about it either. Yes, I come from a place of love but it can also be a place of deafening silence when it comes to healing conversations. There has been little to no mention of my trauma suffered in Detroit Michigan until I released my book in 2019. I know today that this was a coping mechanism to keep me 'safe' and it came out of love...but the reality is the only way to heal is to talk about the uncomfortable truths of our traumas.

Where I'm from and where you're from is uniquely similar and the more we speak about mental health, the faster we normalize the conversation.

CHAPTER NINE
An EAP Saved My Life

WOULD YOU BELIEVE me if I told you that I didn't truly piece together how full circle it was that an EAP (Employee Assistance Program) saved my life? When I wrote 'Tuesdays with Ben' five years ago, I didn't know I would dedicate my next business chapter to speaking about mental health in the workplace. The fact that the EAP at NY Hospital assigned to my Father during my darkest days of addiction would ultimately save my life seems pretty wild right? Then, thirty years later I would go on to speaking about mental health in the workplace?.. it's a lil' freaky deaky. I obtained certification in July of 2023 for Mental Health & Wellness in the Workplace by USF and even then it wasn't clear. I didn't immediately piece everything together, but upon awakening, a profound realization dawned on me. It felt as though everything aligned perfectly, as if I was destined and selected for this purpose.

"Truthfully every road does lead somewhere. For this reason, we should carefully select the paths we take."
-Shirley Desmond Jackson

There is much to be said about the employee health benefits that are offered today in the workplace. I look forward to the day when business owners emphasize the mental health package included in these benefits in unison with physical health. I have spoken to many corporations over the last five years and before I arrive I inquire about these benefits. Nine out of ten times the answer is "I don't know if we have those benefits, I will look into it and get back to you." These resources are vital for HR reps, management, supervisors and hiring managers to understand.

In today's demanding work environments, prioritizing mental health is crucial for employees and employers. When employers openly discuss the mental health benefits they offer, it not only showcases their commitment to employee well being but also helps to normalize conversations about mental health in the workplace. Transparent communication about available resources encourages employees to seek support when needed, fostering a culture of trust and productivity. Moreover, it signals to prospective talent that the company values its employees' holistic health, ultimately leading to higher job satisfaction, retention rates, and overall organizational success.

Imagine the scenario if NY Hospital had not extended its Employee Assistance Program benefits to my Father during one of our family's most challenging times. I was in an alcohol and drug induced blackout 500 miles away and he still had to lead a team of employees every day. His professional role demanded consistent presence, no matter the turmoil unfolding at home. The support from NY Hospital's EAP was not merely a benefit; it was a lifeline to our entire family, through a storm that could have easily overwhelmed us. This resource not only helped him and my family through the most challenging times of his life, it saved MINE! The impact of these employee health benefits kept a family together and now it is my responsibility to spread the word.

Let's start with this question; does mental health live in your home? It would be difficult to encourage mental health in the workplace or anywhere else if it didn't actually live in your own home. This scenario has been running through my mind since my own depression was lifted and the gift of sobriety was bestowed upon me 30 years ago. I was fortunate to piece my life back together as a 21-year-old woman and then navigate my career in the business of medicine for over two decades. The lessons I was learning as a woman in recovery were now being applied to every scenario in business.

When I crawled out of this tumultuous life of addiction and depression, I had an army of support surrounding the climb. I was introduced to my Father's EAP counselor Ben, had the love and support of my family, and a 12-step program that offered a design for living. I was slowly able to encourage a life of mental health that transcended from my home to the workplace but that came after a serious housecleaning.

This process of 'cleaning house' was long and

full of life lessons I choose not to learn again. I had to take a serious look at the people I was surrounding myself with and then determine why I was attracting them in my life. Yes, why was I inviting toxicity into my life and in the workplace even though I was now sober? It is certainly not an overnight process but each moral inventory I took benefitted my quality of life.

I had many issues to overcome as a result of the trauma I endured within my addiction so this was going to be a long housecleaning. There are big and small changes we can all make to ensure mental health lives inside our home and extends to the outside. Let's start with taking a look at who we are surrounding ourselves with on a daily basis. If you find yourself spending any amount of time with a human being that negatively impacts your mental health, you are putting yourself at risk. Turns out it's true that who you surround yourself with is who you are so take a moment to consider how that looks for you today. Yes, that means your family, friends, relationship, co-workers, board members, and your boss.

Now I would like for you to consider how

you are treating your body. I am by no means a clinician, but studies have proven for centuries that diet and exercise directly improve your health and that includes our brain health. Spending time in nature and listening to positive information via a podcast or audible book can also encourage your mental health without spending a co-pay. I am 100% behind talk therapy and all others forms of self-improvement via a mental health professional. In fact, I encourage it if you still think you might have all the answers.

I am a firm believer that our environment can have a huge impact on our mental health. Natural sunlight and bright spaces within our homes and offices can shift our mindset. If you love flowers, plants and music, they can certainly contribute to brightening up a dark day. Let's not forget about our fur-babies and the incredible emotional support they can provide to our well-being. These are all practical suggestions but imperative to consider if you or someone else in your home suffers from depression, anxiety, and beyond.

It is my hope that you will do your own self-reflection and pinpoint places you can improve. It is best to do some internal work before expecting a happy and joyous life at home and in business. If you lead an organization and are unaware of how you can improve the mental health of your company it is past the time you get educated. Yes, as the leader of a company it is your responsibility to offer a physical & mental safe space for your team to reside. I do not pull any punches when it comes to the mental health of your employees, as life is way too fragile. Hopefully we all learned through the pandemic pause and now take necessary actions to live your best life inside and outside of the home.

If you're a business owner, executive, manager, or supervisor find out immediately what mental health benefits are included in your insurance package. It is your responsibility to openly share these life saving resources with your team unapologetically. You can and will save a life. I certainly empathize that not all business owners can afford to offer insurance but there are a multitude of free resources that I will include at the end of this book. Please be sure to share them with your team.

If you're worried about potential job

repercussions for asking about mental health benefits, it's important to proceed cautiously. This is a REAL concern and I empathize with your hesitation. Firstly, know your rights under relevant laws and regulations regarding workplace discrimination based on mental health. Seek confidential support from trusted colleagues, mentors, or external resources like therapists. Familiarize yourself with your company's policies on mental health benefits and consider scheduling a private meeting with HR or a manager to discuss your inquiries discreetly. Obviously not all HR/managers are trusted resources so I would encourage you to document any conversations for your records and explore anonymous feedback channels if available. Remember, prioritizing your mental health is paramount, and there are resources available to support you both within and outside of your workplace.

CHAPTER TEN
The Deafening Silence

NOW WANT TO elaborate on how strongly I feel about having this conversation about mental health in life, and in business. In chapter eight I shared the talk "Where I'm From" because it seems as though saying the words mental health are littered by unnecessary shame and limiting beliefs. The knowledge I have gained by unmet teachers mentioned earlier have truly expanded my yearning to break the cycles of generational trauma. Since I have not birthed my own children, I only have this vehicle of writing to impart my learned wisdom. Listening to all of you has played a huge part in my own healing journey and helped me to dig even deeper. Unfortunately, these last five years of living out loud has not yet penetrated within some of my deepest relationships. This generational trauma that I've come to learn about has been passed down through my family and still cuts deep. A deafening silence remains even after releasing my memoir and I have no control over it today. The fear living behind the root of the core wounds remains in scornful silence.

It took working on myself for 3 decades to scratch the surface so at least I know there is hope. I also know that every time I sit down with the intention to heal, I am not just working on myself; I'm doing work for all those who came before and all those who come after me. The way you live your life matters, not just to you but also to your entire family line. "When pain becomes art" is a phrase that describes how people use trauma as a way to cope with pain and reclaim control. An artistic delivery like the song "When Scars Become Art" by Gatton can help us move past lasting scars of trauma by creating incredible music. These wounds can inspire some of the most beautiful paintings and bring pieces of art that offers profound messages.

"I've heard it said that beauty is when scars become art."

-Gatton

I have learned so much over the last few years and now understand that intergenerational trauma refers to the transmission of unresolved trauma and it's psychological, emotional, and physical effects from one generation to another. It can manifest in various ways through addiction, depression, hording, obesity, unhealthy relationships, people pleasing, and many other harmful behaviors. Although it can be greeted with dismissive blame at times, acknowledging and actively addressing these wounds are the only way to break free from it's influence on future generations.

Today we have an abundance of resources to heal these wounds but it must be met with a willingness to do the work. Hence why I use the term deafening silence so often. I witness pain inflicted on so many people around me and instead of seeking a safe space to heal it is mostly met with "I'm fine." There is a deep shame passed down from generations that **sounds** like this: get over it, that was the past, move on, other people have been through worse, it wasn't that bad, I'm fine now, pull yourself up by your bootstraps, you weren't beaten ... any sound familiar? Now that you know what it sounds like consider what it **looks** like? Anger, resentment, jealousy, alcoholism, addiction, depression, fear of looking stupid, anxiety, OCD, emotional outbursts and so on.

> *"If it's hysterical, it's historical"*
> *-Lori Gottlieb*

Have you ever asked yourself why it's so hard to communicate your vulnerable feelings to another? Is this a learned behavior? Did you come from a family that walked on eggshells and internalized pain? Do you say sorry every time you cry in public? Have you ever felt safe sharing your pain with those closest to you? Do you cry alone more than with a trusted friend or family member? We pass on a mess sometimes ...we're flawed humans...but acknowledging it and making a commitment to change benefits everyone around us.

Why is it so hard to have these uncomfortable

conversations surrounding mental health in life and in business?

Having uncomfortable conversations about mental health can be challenging due to the obvious stigma, fear of repercussions, lack of understanding, cultural & generational factors, and the perception of weakness. It all leads to fear of judgment and obviously employees fear they'll be passed over for opportunities, which definitely deters staff from speaking up. Furthermore, expressing vulnerability can be challenging, especially in environments that prioritize professionalism. If our families consistently make jokes regarding mental health issues, that deafening silence gets real loud for the one suffering. There's often this perception that acknowledging mental health struggles is a sign of weakness, further discouraging us from opening up. In business settings, these challenges can be compounded by concerns about productivity and performance. However, fostering a culture of openness and support around mental health can ultimately benefit both individuals and organizations by promoting trust, and employee well-being. It will always be the responsibility of leadership to set the tone and promote mental health awareness initiatives.

There are simply too many people struggling in the world to remain silent anymore. If you are reading this book today there is a very good chance someone you know and love has died by suicide and or an overdose. It is time we normalize this conversation so we don't lose anymore loved ones. We need to cultivate environments that encourage emotional expression and vulnerability, where people feel comfortable embracing their feelings and tears without judgment. Suppressing discussions about suicide or overdose within our families only perpetuates the silence and fails to honor the life that was lost.

When children witness a lack of healthy communication about pain and loss, it can instill in them a belief that such emotions are taboo or unacceptable. This can hinder their ability to process their own feelings and lead to difficulties in expressing themselves and seeking support when needed. If we strive to empower future generations and foster open conversations about mental health and emotional distress, we win. Suppressing struggles with mental health and addiction within families fosters a culture of silence and this is so loud in our world today it's actually deafening.

Mocking therapy or resisting it ourselves sends a damaging message to future generations, implying that seeking help for mental health issues is shameful or weak. This can deter them from seeking support when needed and instill a cycle of untreated mental health challenges. Demonstrating a double standard by encouraging others to seek help while you have a hard time putting down your phone or barrel through a gallon of ice cream in front of the TV sends conflicting messages. It undermines the importance of consistency and can confuse others about healthy habits and responsible behavior about a life of wellness.

Young men, in particular, who are told by their families that seeking therapy signifies weakness, are likely to develop harmful beliefs. They might come to view vulnerability as shameful, adopting the belief that they must manage their emotions independently. This mindset can potentially exacerbate existing mental health issues. Additionally, they may struggle to develop healthy coping mechanisms, feeling pressure to conform to traditional masculine ideals that prioritize machismo over emotional well-being. We need to do better; our children are watching us more than they're hearing us.

CHAPTER ELEVEN

Isolation to Community; Reflections on AA

JUST LEFT MY Sunday morning Alcoholics Anonymous meeting that I lovingly refer to as 'The Yacht Club.' When the weather is a perfect as it is today in Tampa Bay Florida, I ride my bike to it … today is one of those days. It's April 14th, 2024 and days like this remind me why I am so in love with where I live. I guess I should also mention that nicknames are a thing in AA so let's just leave it at that for now. There's a lot of long-term sobriety here, something I crave as I stay on this broken road to mental health. The things I am attracted to in life over these last 3 decades have shifted tremendously and I thought this was a good place to tell you about it.

The parallel to my early recovery was surrounding myself with people who were sober that same amount of time as me…makes sense right? When my depression lifted after my first year of recovery I found the most wonderful young people trudging this same road of happy destiny. We were all climbing out of the rubble and challenged with so many of the same issues. I know the friends put in my life at that time were exactly what I needed, they saved my life. One of many gifts I received in early recovery was a beautiful group of men and women in their early 20's getting sober. We went on trips together, met each other at meetings, went to the diner for fellowship, and talked on the phone daily. These friends carried me through some of the most challenging days of early recovery. One of those friends died from an overdose on June 10th, 2021. She would have celebrated her 60th birthday this year but sadly, she was taken way too soon from this disease of addiction. I have lost touch with 90% of those friends I got sober, especially because I left NY 20 years ago. When I got the call about my friend, it really shook me. An incredible deep feeling of sadness lived within me for many days as I reminisced of how smart, funny, and breath-takingly beautiful she was. She lovingly referred to me as 'Gabone,' although the urban dictionary says it's an Italian slang for crude person. Hmm. Seems fitting as I was pretty crude in early recovery and can still teeter on raw and unrefined even today.

She left a mark in my heart that lives inside me today. Her soul seemed tortured because she felt love so deeply…we use to light candles and read from the daily reflections book 'Language of Letting Go' by Melody Beattie. On the day of her passing, the reading unfolded like this:

"Responsibility"

Self care means taking responsibility for ourselves. Taking responsibility for ourselves includes assuming our true responsibilities to others.

Sometimes, when we begin recovery, we're worn down from feeling responsible for so many other people. Learning that we need only take responsibility for ourselves may be such a great relief that, for a time, we disown our responsibilities to others.

The goal in recovery is to find the balance: we take responsibility for ourselves, and we identify our true responsibilities to others.

This may take some sorting through, especially if we have functioned for years on distorted notions about our responsibilities to others. We may be responsible to one person as a friend or as an employee; to another person, we're responsible as an employer or as a spouse. With each person, we have certain responsibilities. When we tend to those true responsibilities, we'll find balance in our life.

We are also learning that while others aren't responsible for us, they are accountable to us in certain ways.

We can learn to discern our true responsibilities for ourselves, and to others. We can allow others to be responsible for themselves and expect them to be appropriately responsible to us.

We'll need to be gentle with ourselves while we learn.

Today, I will strive for clear thinking about my actual responsibilities to others. I will assume these responsibilities as part of taking care of myself."

-From The Language of Letting Go by Melody Beattie ©1990, Hazelden Foundation.

Understanding the crucial importance of self-care in taking responsibility for ourselves may not be fully realized by many of us yet. It took almost 25 years for me to fully embrace this notion and I unapologetically put myself first today. I am grateful to have remained open to the many mentors that have come before me to amplify this message.

Now, back to the meaning behind the chapter title. When you enter into a 12-step program, the word 'isolation' is said daily, loud and proud. We have been using this word for over 80 years to drive home the importance of fellowship and community. There was a time I resented hearing someone ask, "Sharon, are you isolating?" Now, I'm profoundly thankful that this concern is deeply ingrained within me. The word isolation permeated the world, becoming a prevalent topic in the media and everyday conversations as the pandemic unfolded. I began to consider how powerful this free life-saving program I have been a part of for 30 years saved so many of us in the pandemic and yet tragically increased the amounts of overdoses and suicides. In 2023, the Surgeon General called attention to the public health crisis of loneliness, isolation, and lack of connection in our country stating that disconnection affects our mental, physical, and societal health. He said lacking connection increases the risk for premature death and it's comparable to smoking daily.

For those fellow friends of Bill out there (Google the reference) you know this to be factual and true. The one thing I have struggled the most with through my years of sobriety is staying away from isolation. I've already elaborated on how I practice 'opposite action' because everything in my brain screams, "ISOLATE!" I spent six entire months in isolation during my crippling depression when I was 21 years old. The only times I went outside was when someone was dragging me to an AA meeting

The Broken OPEN Road To Mental Health

or I was taking the train into Manhattan to see my EAP counselor, Ben. I am 100% on board with the Surgeon General, I wonder if he consulted AA members in the research?! That said, I truly felt for those about to embark on sobriety in 2020 and was heartbroken to know they wouldn't have the community so desperately needed in those early days of abstinence. This prompted me to hop on the ZOOM train and start a weekly online meeting called Recovery Journey to Mental Wellness' that is still going strong today. Trust me, I'm not one to start a meeting but I have since began two over the last 5 years. I remember my dear friend Jimmy Marino, that has since passed on, telling me if doesn't exist, create it. The next meeting that didn't exist in my community was a weekly in-person woman run Big Book Study. I am proud to say these meetings are still going strong and run by my sponsee and dear friend Kelli. This concept of "the spirit of rotation" holds significant truth. I can't wait to see who she passes it on to next.

An AA pamphlet published in 2018 was brought to my attention by my dear friend Nancy. We read from this pamphlet weekly at our Saturday morning ZOOM meeting and so many have found solace in this safe space. I believe in my heart and soul if Bill W. (Founder of AA) was alive today, he would have integrated a mental health component to the program. If you have done any deep dives on Bill Wilson you know that he suffered for years with depression. We do evolve and hopefully this program of recovery that saves my life every day will follow suit in the near future.

CHAPTER TWELVE
HEALERS

Little Sharon wanted to be a therapist. Sober Sharon wanted to be a therapist. Business Sharon became a COACHultant. Let me explain… we'll get back to that made up word soon.

Mom referred to me as 'Dear Abby' as a child because all my friends came to me with their problems. I loved offering advice, even when you didn't ask for it. I have simply always been fascinated with the psychology of humans but never had a desire to obtain that degree. Instead, I became the boss in my early twenties and remained as such until turning 40. Then, I got paid to solve problems in business for physicians, therapists, business owners, and beyond.

Being a boss and being a therapist share several common elements, even though their primary roles and contexts are obviously very different. Both roles require strong listening and empathy skills, as a good boss listens to their employees' concerns and challenges, while a therapist listens empathetically to their clients' problems and experiences. Building trust is crucial in both positions; employees need to trust that their boss has their best interests at heart, just as clients need to feel safe and confident in their therapist's support and confidentiality. Guidance and support are also key aspects, with bosses providing direction on tasks and career development, and therapists guiding clients through emotional and psychological challenges. Both roles involve conflict resolution, whether it's managing workplace disputes or helping clients resolve internal conflicts and relationship issues. Additionally, both bosses and therapists are tasked with motivating and encouraging growth, recognizing achievements, and fostering development in their team members or clients.

At the end of 2023, I made the decision to focus my final efforts in business doing exactly what I love until the day I retire. I'm currently a keynote speaker and a business/life COACHultant. I'm literally sitting in a hotel room right now writing my last two chapters the night before getting on stage to speak to business owners. It's a life I do not take for granted and simultaneously think is batshit because I was literally homeless and addicted 30 years ago. Anyway, a COACHultant is a hybrid role that combines the skills and approaches of both a coach and a consultant. I blend personalized, developmental coaching with strategic consulting. My role focuses on personal development by helping clients enhance their skills, mindset, and potential, while empowering them to achieve personal and professional goals through encouragement and accountability. I also provide expert advice in business strategy, problem-solving, and offer actionable solutions. By integrating coaching and consulting, I can address both immediate business needs and long-term personal development. I also love confusing people to think I have something to do with Coachella.

Having 30 years of sobriety and being a survivor of depression, combined with my extensive experience as both a boss and a business owner, I make an exceptional life coach as a wounded healer for several reasons.

Overcoming significant personal challenges such as addiction and depression has given me a deep sense of empathy for clients facing similar struggles. My firsthand experience provides a profound understanding of the emotional and psychological hurdles that they may encounter, making my guidance more relatable and impactful. My journey of thirty years of sobriety and surviving depression offers hope to inspire my clients by showing them that recovery and success are possible, even after enduring significant hardships.

With 20 years of experience as a boss and 10 years running my own business, I have honed leadership, management, and problem-solving skills. These skills are invaluable in life coaching, where guiding clients through personal and professional challenges is essential. Running a business for a decade has provided me with practical insights into entrepreneurship and strategic planning, which can help my clients navigate their own business ventures or career paths more effectively.

As a wounded healer, my authenticity and

credibility are enhanced by my life experiences. Clients are likely to trust and respect a healer who has successfully navigated similar struggles and emerged stronger. My diverse background allows me to take a holistic approach to coaching, addressing both personal and professional aspects of my clients' lives. This comprehensive perspective ensures that they receive well-rounded support and guidance.

Now that you have a little insight into my love for all things therapy, coaching, and business strategizing, let's talk about healers. I have a deep affection and preference for a wounded healer for my own life to help me today. I can't help but question why so many healers (therapists, doctors, psychiatrists, psychologists, and beyond) don't use their healed wounds as superpowers. There have been countless clients that have crossed my path that I sit in amazement about their why as to not share their past to help someone's future. On the contrary, I also deeply respect that not everyone wants to be vulnerable and fears what revealing their past lives might implicate, but dare I say more people struggling would be attracted to this human struggle? Truthfully, a large piece of me wants to offer this feedback to you reader, because I absolutely know people like me that have struggled deeply desire identification. For over 80 years now, FREE 12 step programs have offered grace to millions of people based largely on lack of judgment and simply relating to another human being.

I also want to express my thoughts about the enormous amount of choices we have today to heal. It doesn't have to be therapy or 12 step recovery but it has to be something. Healing encompasses a wide range of modalities that address physical, emotional, mental, and spiritual aspects of well being. Alternative practices like acupuncture, massage therapy, herbal medicine, and nutrition play significant roles in maintaining physical and mental health.

Emotional healing can also include art and music therapy for expressing and processing emotions.

There are also so many forms of therapy including cognitive behavioral therapy, trauma therapy, family therapy, sex therapy, mindfulness and meditation practices, and actually a simple walk in the park could help. Spiritual healing practices are good for the soul and come in many forms. Yoga, breathing exercises, meditation, laughter, music, dancing, traveling…all remedies promote overall well-being.

Social healing involves support groups and community-building that fosters a sense of belonging and support. Please understand that community is crucial for our mental health because it provides the emotional support we all need to survive. Being part of a community helps reduce feelings of loneliness and offers encouragement during difficult times. Social interactions within a community contribute to us feeling valued and understood. Additionally, community involvement encourages healthy behaviors and provides opportunities for personal growth and development, further contributing to overall mental wellness.

In other words, get some damn help please. Stop passing on your shit to future generations and spilling your unhealed trauma on everyone else… yes, this is always what I want to say and since it's MY book, I said it.

Sharon Fekete

If you don't transform your suffering you will transmit it.

— Fr. Richard Rohr

CHAPTER THIRTEEN

Dad, what is this here to teach me?

"You can either break down or you can break open"

-Elizabeth Lasser

HERE IT IS, the last chapter. Personally, there has been much procrastination in writing this chapter. To you, the notion of delaying something by a few weeks may seem trivial. However, in the unique workings of my mind, such a delay feels like an eternity. I wrote my last book in 5 days and then included a bonus chapter, which now honors my favorite number 13. I documented each day of writing on YouTube five years ago and just watched the last day to get inspired to write this one.

I started documenting *this* book on TikTok, sign of the times, but almost (2) months have passed and I'm back in the Tree room. Writing this book has certainly been more challenging. Life is simply different today and although a piece of disappointment in myself creped in, I quickly replaced the thought to remain in a state of flow. Slow down. Take a breath. I don't have to put so much pressure on myself, especially when life has been lifeing all over the place lately.

I mentioned earlier that my Dad was diagnosed with Alzheimer's in 2021 and right now he is in a facility waiting for permanent placement to an Assisted Living Facility. He's been there since February of 2024 and let's just say, it hasn't been easy for anyone in my family. This very personal situation is the reason for my delay; my heart is simply on the cusp of being entirely broken. I'm extra fragile. So, what is this here to teach me? Hell if I know but let's see if we can figure it out together in this chapter. I think you know by now that I am far more a documenter than a writer, I want to bring you with me on this journey of breaking open. Since this chapter will most likely cause the most choking up as I type, I just got up and walked out of the office to change my chair. In my first book I mentioned that one of the Co-Founders of my workspace, The Ring, changed out my chair while I was writing. He didn't know that I was reliving my trauma while I was writing and how monumental that small gesture was at the moment. Since he's not here today and doesn't know I'm writing my book, I got up myself and requested a more comfortable chair. For nostalgia and to simply offer myself some more grace as I channel this pain into words. Well, not only did I get a comfy chair, but my friend Festus brought it to the room for me and we exchanged pleasantries before I got back to writing. Grace accepted real time.

Many things have changed here at The Ring since 2019 but my love for the space and the people remains. I now host an event here based around mental health in the workplace at the end of every month. Simple beauty transpires each time community bonds together and these cherished moments live within the walls of this magical space of wellness. Our shared desire to maximize our human potential and create psychologically safe & courageous spaces lives here at The Ring. I'm honored to work within a space that exemplifies extreme hospitality and unwavering commitment to design, sustainability, and wellness.

Ok…in real time I'm prolonging the pain living in my throat just thinking about the words that will be typed in this chapter. Here's a sneak peak into my brain…I'm also thinking about how I will ever get through recording this for Audible. Somehow, it was easier to write about the pain I endured living through my trauma in the years of my addiction. Thirty years later, my heart is broken open while my Father resides in a facility I'm sure he never could have imagined for himself. Shit, no Kleenex. Ok, I'm back…tears dried.

Yesterday I had a melt down after speaking to one of my favorite clients in NYC, Dr. Cooke. This gift of a woman living on Earth listened to me talk about how great of a singer my Dad is and how his song will forever live inside of me, "Beyond the Sea" by Bobby Darin. I sent her a clip of him singing it and then had an overwhelming desire to call my Uncle Tony in Ireland. I went on

WhatsApp and we talked for 30 minutes as the tears rolled down my face discussing the difficulty of this time in our lives. He recently came from Ireland to visit my Father in this facility with my Aunt Alison and we are forever grateful for the time spent. We reminisced about celebrating Dad's 80th in Dublin, and although he doesn't remember it, those memories will live in our hearts forever. Knowing they were able to spend time with him while he remembers all of us is a beautiful gift.

Talking to Uncle Tony felt like the closest I could get to my Dad as they look and sound so much alike. I made a conscious decision these last few years to never apologize when I'm crying anymore and not to stifle the tears. He heard me cry, that's normal. I no longer want to block the pain and stuff it inside of me, especially since that is how depression presented when I was 21 years old. After our call, I allowed myself a good cry with my dog Charlie Brown & then shared my pain with the biggest gift in my life, my husband Rob. Not too long ago I would have put myself back together and avoided "being a burden" versus sharing the pain with him…no more. Lucky guy gets to hear it ALL now!! This is part of my practice of healing that I actively participate in today. If pain comes knocking on my door I no longer cry in the shower…I let those that love me hear the pain. I remember once believing it was weak to cry, now I feel like a super hero every time I open the flood gates. I have even promised myself to allow it to happen when speaking in front of an audience. This is not something I plan by any means but if it organically comes up, I tell them about the importance of vulnerability

In the words of Dr. Gabor Mate, "trauma is not what happens to us, it's what happens inside of us." I no longer want my body to act as a carrying card member for my pain. Crying in front of others is not only healthy for us but it connects us on a deeper level. I wouldn't say this is a common practice passed down from previous generations but I certainly believe it's time to break the cycle.

CRY!!!

NO APOLOGIZING!!!

SHOW OTHERS YOU ARE HUMAN!!

PLEASE stop saying you're sorry when you're crying, it's the most loving way to heal yourself and

The Broken OPEN Road To Mental Health

those around you. Cry in front of your children, please, and let them see that it's normal to have feelings. Please!

All of us are affected and there are many fractures and cracks in this broken road currently. The pain of witnessing the loss of my Father in real time is affecting all of us in ways I'm quite sure none of us could have ever foreseen. They refer to losing an Alzheimer's patient as 'the long goodbye' and for good reason, it is LONG and it is painful. Each of us individually are experiencing levels of anger, pain, sadness, loneliness, and grief. For the first time in my life, I am not trying to fix it for anyone. I am choosing to apply what I have been taught, this 25 yearlong lesson, to stop trying to fix. THIS is the real work in motion. The overwhelming pull to control, remove pain from others, and fix has been the most difficult lesson to date. Putting myself first and allowing others that I love to experience pain is 100% the hardest. Learning how to let go of guilt and trust in a higher source to work things out is tremendously challenging. Meditation and therapy have been the absolute greatest gifts to me throughout this difficult season and I'm still a work in progress.

I have been a sober woman for the last 30 years. I have done a tremendous amount of work on myself but absolutely nothing has compared to the growth I have felt since releasing my memoir 5 years ago. Finally facing the trauma that lived inside of me has been painful and simultaneously brought me the most peace I have ever known. I have not raged at my husband in years and that suppressed anger that used to visit our family intermittently has finally said goodbye. The suppression of that little girl who endured physical, emotional, and mental torture for 3 years while living in a blackout in Detroit has gone away. This writing has saved my life and is slowly bringing me to the woman I was meant to be. I have fought against the deafening silence that once overwhelmed me, and I am learning to raise my voice more, embracing the power of speaking out. I am deeply thankful for the grace of a slow healing process. Today, I understand that my fragile, recovering mind could not have endured such pain at the tender age of 21.

Though this current pain of witnessing my

Father's decline is gut wrenching, it has also brought me back home to myself. I have recorded many of our bittersweet moments together where he shares his endless love for my mother and my two brothers. He speaks so fondly of the men that worked for and with him at NY hospital and reminds me to never give up, often. His love for Ireland and his family in Dublin is spoken of every time we meet. Even with his failing memory, he has not yet forgotten the pain we all endured as a family when I was living through addiction and depression. He is quick to snap back into gratitude that I made it back home...back home to love.

Life will continue to provide us with opportunities for growth, no matter how much we try to avoid it. I remain hopeful, despite the many fractures and cracks that mark our family's current path. I believe the pain we are experiencing serves a higher purpose, one that we must release and allow to work its transformative power within us. When I'm faced with these challenges today I ask myself ask, what is this here to teach me? Then I listen for the answers in meditation...the solution doesn't always come right away but I know I'm not in charge. When you have faced the dark night of the soul as I have, it's easy to understand on a very spiritual level that nothing is worth losing yourself for... we are here for a reason...let's not waste anymore time.

As I review all the edits my dear friend Alanna provided, I want to say thank you all for following my journey. Michelle, thank you for seeing me and gifting the pen that ultimately shifted my path. I will not offer separate acknowledgements in this book as I did in the last one simply because I'm too sad. Full stop. I want to be entirely authentic with you, reader, and I know on a deep level it's ok not to be ok. I'm not ok right now, but I am light years away from where I once was 30 years ago.

Currently reading 'Broken Open' by Elizabeth Lesser...who knew. I highly encourage you to read it...the whispers flow through every page.

I will forever love you Robert John Fekete, Jr. You have brought me a love I never knew existed. Cooper, you have been one of the greatest gifts in my life and I love you immensely.

Mom, Paul, and Sean... we come from a

foundation of love, the broken road holds the crane. I love you all.

We are all under construction.

Dad always reminds me to stay positive and "be careful" so I will leave you with the same sentiment.

I love you Dad.

I know you will stay in my heart forever.

I will see you again, somewhere beyond the sea.

Printed in the USA
CPSIA information can be obtained
at www.ICGtesting.com
CBHW070745180824
13253CB00059B/1034